Atkins Diet:

4 Weeks To Cracked Weight Loss, Strongest Energy And Better Your Life

Lose Up 1 Pound Per Day

By Jeremy Torres

Owlprince Publishing Limited

D1530508

Disclaimer Notice:

Please note the information contained within this document is for educational and entertainment purposes only. Every attempt has been made to provide accurate, up to date and reliable, complete information. No warranties of any kind are expressed or implied. Readers acknowledge that the author is not engaging in the rendering of legal, financial, medical or professional advice.

By reading this document, the reader agrees that under no circumstances are we responsible for any losses, direct or indirect, which are incurred as a result of the use of information contained within this document, including, but not limited to, —errors, omissions, or inaccuracies.

Contents

Introduction

Firstly I would like to congratulate you and thank you for choosing this book: " Atkins Diet: 4 Weeks To Cracked Weight Loss, Strongest Energy And Better Your Life- Lose Up 1 Pound Per Day (Including The Very Best Atkins Diet Recipe)".

Do you feel like you haven't been blessed with the best fat burning genetics? Does food seem to go straight to your problem areas like your belly, bum and thighs? Do you feel like you've tried every diet known to man but the weight keeps coming back?

What If I told you that you could lose weight, feel better, look better, have more energy, reduce pain, boost your sex drive, prevent disease ··· and best of all you'll still be able to still eat some of the foods you crave the most and still experience a slimmer body? Atkins Diet will be your right answer...

Created by a well-renowned cardiologist, Robert C. Atkins in the year 1972, the core structure of this Atkins diet will influence you to cut down carbohydrate intake and focus more on foods containing fats and protein.

By following a low carb high fat & protein Atkins Diet, it won't only help you to trim down your weight, but will also help you to stay healthy and fit for the rest of your life.

Below is some of the benefits you will get from this diet of this book:

1. Drop in blood sugar and insulin levels

2. Rapid Weight loss

3. Lower the risk of cancer

4. Better skin and reduce acne

5. Reduction of appetite

6. Lower your blood pressure

7. Sleep well and get up timely & easily

8. Better mood

9. Be longevity

......

This book suit for people of any weight, any body type or shape. Through my work, I've helped thousands of people achieve their health and fat loss goals, and I share everything I know in my books.

I've already made this book to lead anyone from new comer to professional. So you can know what foods to eat and what to avoid, helping nourish properly and support long lasting fat loss, anti-aging, boundless natural energy and a better mood.

What will you find in this book?

1. Origins of the Atkins Diet dating back to the 1970s

2. The study about using Atkins Diet for weight loss & health

3. Benefits about Atkins diet

4. Super tips for your success of Atkins diet

5. 4 Weeks Easy-To-Follow Atkins Diet Meal Plan with Breakfast, Lunch, Dinner, snack and dessert

6. Foods to be eat and to be avoided

7. 40 easy to make and delicious recipes support your Atkins Diet journey

8. Each meal have detailed nutrition value and step by step procedure, even an idiot can make all of these flavored recipes

9. And much much more!

All methods in this book are so easy and simple, and so powerful to you. That it will maybe sound like too unbelievable when you read it at first time. This Amazing Fat Destroying method will give you an absolute body changeover without any supplements, workouts or high price ineffective pills. Hope you will get what you want from this amazing book!

God Bless!

Jeremy Torres

Chapter 1:

Getting To Know The Secret Behind Atkins Diet

A brief overview of Atkins Diet

Having its origins set in the early 1970s, Atkins Diet is an immensely popular method of losing weight that was first established by cardiologist Robert C. Atkins during the year 1972. The primary objective of this diet plan is to lower the carbohydrate intake of the body while putting a bigger emphasis on fats and proteins.

Following an appropriately oriented Atkins Diet, you won't only be able to establish a much healthier physique by putting your excess weight to rest. You will also be able to achieve a much more balanced and organized lifestyle.

Generally speaking, If you fall upon any of the following categories, then you might be interested in going on an Atkins Diet

- If you enjoy the different types of food which represent Atkins Diet
- You are looking for a diet where you want to keep your carbohydrate intake in check

- Want to substantially alter your eating habits and transcend to a healthier lifestyle
- You are facing some medical issues which might be tackled by following Atkins Diet

However, if you decide to embark on a journey of Atkins Diet, you can check up with your nutritionist/physician firstly to make sure that you don't have any medical issues which might negatively impact your health.

The different phases of Atkins Diet

The basic procedure followed by an Atkins Diet will require you to go through four distinct steps, each of which has specific requirements that will help you achieve maximum results. The breakdown of the four stages are as follows

Phase 1: The first phase is known as the "Induction" phase where you are required to cut out the maximum amount of Carbohydrates from your day to day diet. Restricting yourself to just 20g of Carbs per day, which should mainly come from vegetables. Here your main focus should be on green vegetables, and as for protein, you might opt for fish, poultry, shellfish, and eggs and so on. While oil or fat are not that much affected here, you should try to keep yourself away from sugary baked goods, bread, pasta, grain, and alcohol.

Phase 2: The second phase is known as "Balancing." Here you are to take a minimum carbohydrates of 12-15g which should come from foundation vegetables. After which you can slowly revert to some more nutrient rich carbohydrates, so as long as you are losing weight. It is important to stay in this phase until you are just 4.5kg away from your main goal

Phase 3: The third phase is Pre-Maintenance. Here you are going to want to continue increasing the amount of nutrient-rich carb intake which will comprise of starchy vegetables, whole grains, and some fruits. You should keep increasing 10g of carb per week to your diet and keep in mind that you should not increase your intake too high in case that you start gaining weight.

Phase 4: The final phase is the "Lifetime Maintenance" phase. Once you have achieved your weight, then from now on you are just required to keep following the specified diet.

How does Atkins Diet Work?

Before understanding how Atkins Diet works, a little word on the human body's metabolism function is required. The key here is to know that our body uses two different sources of "Fuel" if you will see which it uses for energy. It can either go for sugar or it can either go for fat.

When you are on a regular diet, what it does is to force you to reduce your calories intake. While you remain high in the sugar (carbohydrate).

So, what happens here is that when the body requires more energy, it breaks down this sugar instead of the fat.

Alternatively, when you are on a Atkins Diet. Since the carbohydrate intake is drastically limited, the body starts to use up fat as a source of energy, which in return results in the body losing weight rapidly.

And this is not just word of mouth! More than 80 different and extremely thorough clinical studies have already proven this point!

Atkins and weight loss

I am pretty sure that the first target for you while reading this book is to know about how soon you will be able to lose your weight by using Atkins Diet.

Well, you should understand that weight loss through Atkins maybe not very fast as different people have diferent body type or conditions.

Maybe when it comes to you, the speed of losing fat slower and gradually. By reading this book cannot make you cut your fat rapidly, but it will give you a stable and continuous fat loss and give you a healthier body by taking action following Atkins Diet.

When you first start off your diet during your Induction phase, you should expect a weight loss of somewhere around 6-10 pound in the first week.

After that, during the following weeks, you should expect a weight loss clocking around 1-3 pound per week.

And finally, once you have entered your pre-maintenance phase, you should expect about 1 or 2 pound per week.

Benefits of Atkins Diet

You may be interested in following an Atkins Diet just for weight loss, but you should also know that there's a lot more to Atkins Diet than just weight loss!

- The first and foremost, obviously it will help you to lose your weight!
- It will contribute to deal with Epilepsy
- The low carb atkins diet will contribute to mitigate any acid-related problem
- Atkins Diet will contribute to improve your skin conditions and reduce ACNE
- This diet will help you to minimize the amount of headache you experience from
- A low carb diet such as this will also help you to reduce the risk of undergoing any cardiovascular disease
- With reduces obesity and better health conditions, Atkins Diet will also help you to prevent yourself from being affected by cancer
- This diet will also contribute to aging women to tackle PCOS syndrome.

Tips for a successful Atkins Diet

With this following tips, you can very quickly touch the goal to fat loss in following your Atkins Diet!

- Make sure know what kind of food you are eating, and you know how the different phases of Atkins works
- Experiment and find the Atkins Diet routine suitable for you
- Keep count of your Carbohydrates
- Be calculative and sensible when choosing your portions
- Make sure you are not starving! Eat accordingly, but in small portions and low carbs
- Every meal should have at least a minimal amount of protein
- Try to opt for food which is made of natural fat
- Stay away from sugar
- Eat lots of vegetables
- Make sure to drink lots of water

- If possible, then take daily vitamin supplements to make sure that your body is not going through any deficiency
- Just sitting down and dieting won't do any good to you! Move out there and try to get some physical exercise as well
- Make sure to keep track of your success rate which will further help encouraging you to keep moving forward

Make sure to avoid the following foods whenever possible!

- Sugary drinks such as fruit juice, cake, ice cream
- Grains such as rye, barley, wheat
- Vegetable oils such as corn oil, soybean oil, cottonseed oil
- Food with "hydrogenated" ingredients
- Foods labeled "Diet Food "
- High Carb vegetables as Carrots or turnips (This should be avoided only during your induction phases)

- High Carb Fruits such as apples, bananas, oranges (Again, this should only be avoided during induction phases)
- Starches such as potatoes (Avoid only in induction phase)
- Legumes such as beans and lentils (only during induction phase)

Try to go for these foods

- Meats such as pork, beef, chicken, lamb and also bacon
- Fatty Fish such as trout, tilapia, salmon
- Eggs that are rich in Omega 3
- Low Carb vegetables as spinach, kale, asparagus
- Full-Fat Dairy products such as Butter, cream, yogurt
- Nuts and seeds including macadamia nuts, almonds, walnuts and so on
- Healthy fat including extra virgin olive oil, avocado, and coconut oil

Chapter 2: Phase Wise Meal Plan

As you now know, instead of going for weeks, Atkins Diet requires you to go through different "Phases" of the diet. In this chapter, I will be outlining a rough meal plan of all the four phases which you could follow up until you have reached a certain level of your goal.

For phase 1, your target should be to keep your carb intake under 20 grams per day and go for high fat/high protein meals with an assortment of low carb vegetables. It is normally necessary to continue this phase for 2 weeks in order to jump start your weight loss.

Phase 1 Shopping List

- Salt as required
- Sucralose based Sweetener
- Cinnamon
- Unsalted Butter Stick
- Low Carb Baking Mix
- Tap Water
- Almond Meal Flour
- High Fiber Coconut Flour (Organic)

- Cinnamon
- Baking Powder
- Egg
- Extra Virgin Olive Oil
- Butter filled boneless pork loin chops
- Blue Cheese
- Bacon slices
- Garlic
- Ground Pepper as required
- Fresh Parsley
- Parmesan Cheese
- Softened Butter
- Red Tomato
- Cilantro
- Red Onion
- Jalapeno Popper
- Avocado
- Mayonnaise
- Lemon Juice
- Basil
- Onion Powder
- Celery Salt
- Tilapia Fillet
- Tamari Soybean Sauce

- Worcestershire Sauce
- Canola Vegetable Oil
- Pork Chop with Center Loin and Bone In
- Cayenne Powder
- Yellow Mustard Seed
- Bone-in Chicken Wing

Phase 1 Meal Plan

Day One

(Totals: Calorie: 625; fat: 52.3g; net carbs: 15.5g ; Protein: 53.9)

Breakfast:

Delicious Almond and Coconut Muffin (Calorie: 207; Fat: 16.8; Carbohydrate: 3.5g; Dietary Fiber: 3g; Protein:9.7g)

Snack

Greenful Avocado Salsa (Calorie: 71; Fat: 5.3g; Carbohydrate: 3.3g; Protein: 1.1g)

Lunch

Healthy Broiled Up Tilapia Parmesan (Calorie: 224; Fat: 12.8g: Carbohydrate: 0.8g; Protein: 25.4g)

Dinner

Tender Baked Tamari Lemon Pork Chops (Calorie: 149; Fat: 8g: Carbohydrate: 4g; Protein: 15.2g)

Dessert

Lightly Sweet Chocolate Brownie Drops (Calorie: 104; Fat: 9.4g: Carbohydrate: 3.9g; Protein: 2.5g)

Day Two

(Total: Calories: 1302; fat: 75.5g; net carbs: 14.3g; protein:50.1)

Breakfast:

Fantastic Atkins Pie Crust (Calorie: 193; Fat: 13.6g: Carbohydrate: 2.5g; Protein: 14.8g)

Snack

Bony Chicken Wingettes (Calorie: 276; Fat: 18.5g: Carbohydrate: 3.4g; Protein: 22g)

Lunch

Asian Beef Salad (Calorie: 295; Fat: 13.3g: Carbohydrate: 10.4g; Protein: 29.5gg)

Dinner

Dreamy Cali Mac And Cheese (Calorie: 320; Fat: 27g: Carbohydrate: 5.6g; Protein: 11.4g)

Dessert

Unexpected Baked Pear Fan (Calorie: 80; Fat: 3g: Carbohydrate: 11.5g; Protein: 0.4g)

Day Three

(Totals: Calorie: 911; fat: 70.8g; net carbs: 17g ; Protein: 58.7g)

Breakfast:

Buttery Soft Cuisine Waffles (Calorie: 193; Fat: 9; Carbohydrate: 5.9; Dietary Fiber: 1.9g; Protein:9.7g)

Snack

Magnificent Artichoke With Three Cheese (Calorie: 57; Fat: 14g: Carbohydrate: 3g; Protein: 4g)

Lunch

Luscious Crust Less Quiche Lori Lane (Calorie: 224; Fat: 12.8g: Carbohydrate: 0.8g; Protein: 25.4g)

Dinner

Tender Baked Tamari Lemon Pork Chops (Calorie: 149; Fat: 8g: Carbohydrate: 4g; Protein: 15.2g)

Dessert

Fantastic Caramelized Pear Custard (Calorie: 310; Fat: 27g: Carbohydrate: 4.2g; Protein: 4.4g)

Day Four

(Total: Calories: 1033; fat: 82.9g; net carbs: 19.6g; protein:48.3g)

Breakfast:

Delicious Almond and Coconut Muffin (Calorie: 207 ; Fat: 16.8g ; net carbs: 3.5g ; Protein: 9.7g)

Snack

Berryful Black Berry Peach Compote (Calorie: 35; Fat: 0.2g: Carbohydrate: 4.2g; Protein: 0.5g)

Lunch

Succulent Pan Fried Tuna Patty (Calorie: 367; Fat: 29.3g: Carbohydrate: 2.4g; Protein:24.2g)

Dinner

Dreamy Cali Mac And Cheese (Calorie: 320; Fat: 27g: Carbohydrate: 5.6g; Protein: 11.4g

Dessert

Lightly Sweet Chocolate Brownie Drops (Calorie: 104 ; Fat: 9.4g: Carbohydrate: 3.9g; Protein: 2.5g)

Day Five

(Totals: Calorie: 1275; fat: 88.7g; net carbs: 18.9g ; Protein: 84.4g)

Breakfast

Finely Baked Egg Asparagus (Calorie: 471; Fat: 40g; Carbohydrate: 5.6gg; Dietary Fiber: 4g; Protein: 20.8g)

Snack

Fantastic Atkins Cinnamon Pie Crust (Calorie: 193; Fat: 13.6g: Carbohydrate: 2.5g; Protein: 14.8g)

Lunch

Healthy Broiled Up Tilapia Parmesan (Calorie: 224; Fat: 12.8g: Carbohydrate: 0.8g; Protein: 25.4g)

Dinner

Tender Baked Tamari Lemon Pork Chops (Calorie: 149; Fat: 8g: Carbohydrate: 4g; Protein: 15.2g)

Dessert

Classical Apple Tart (Calorie: 238; Fat: 14.3g: Carbohydrate: 6g; Protein: 8.2g)

Day Six

(Total: Calories: 1439g; fat: 100.5g; net carbs: 11.9g; protein:77.2)

Breakfast:

Fantastic Atkins Pie Crust (Calorie: 193; Fat: 13.6g: Carbohydrate: 2.5g; Protein: 14.8g)

Snack

Indian Chicken Curry (Calorie: 413; Fat: 22.1g: Carbohydrate: 1g; Protein: 49.1g)

Lunch

Healthy Blue Cheese, Bacon and Chive Stuffed Up Pork Chops (Calorie: 394; Fat: 26.3g: Carbohydrate: 2g; Protein:0.3g)

Dinner

Dreamy Cali Mac And Cheese (Calorie: 320; Fat: 27g: Carbohydrate: 5.6g; Protein: 11.4g)

Dessert

Chocolaty Chocolate Cream Frosty (Calorie: 119 ; Fat: 11.5g: Carbohydrate: 0.8g; Protein: 1.6g)

Day Seven

(Totals: Calorie: 755; fat: 52.3g; net carbs: 15.5g ; Protein: 53.9)

Breakfast:

Delicious Almond and Coconut Muffin (Calorie: 207; Fat: 16.8; Carbohydrate: 3.5g; Dietary Fiber: 3g; Protein:9.7g)

Snack

Greenful Avocado Salsa (Calorie: 71; Fat: 5.3g: Carbohydrate: 3.3g; Protein: 1.1g)

Lunch

Healthy Broiled Up Tilapia Parmesan (Calorie: 224; Fat: 12.8g: Carbohydrate: 0.8g; Protein: 25.4g)

Dinner

Tender Baked Tamari Lemon Pork Chops (Calorie: 149; Fat: 8g: Carbohydrate: 4g; Protein: 15.2g)

Dessert

Lightly Sweet Chocolate Brownie Drops (Calorie: 104; Fat: 9.4g: Carbohydrate: 3.9g; Protein: 2.5g)

Upon completing your second week in phase 1, you should move ahead to phase 2 and continue following this until you are just about 4.5-5kg away from your goal. This phase will primarily follow your previous diet, with an included amount of more nuts and vegetables.

Phase 2 Shopping List

- Salt as required
- Sucralose based Sweetener
- Cinnamon
- Unsalted Butter Stick
- Low Carb Baking Mix
- Tap Water
- Almond Meal Flour
- High Fiber Coconut Flour (Organic)
- Cinnamon
- Baking Powder
- Egg
- Extra Virgin Olive Oil
- Butter filled boneless pork loin chops
- Blue Cheese

- Bacon slices
- Garlic
- Ground Pepper as required
- Fresh Parsley
- Parmesan Cheese
- Softened Butter
- Red Tomato
- Cilantro
- Red Onion
- Jalapeno Popper
- Avocado
- Mayonnaise
- Lemon Juice
- Basil
- Onion Powder
- Celery Salt
- Greek Yogurt
- Atkins Peanut Butter Granola Bar
- Large Strawberries
- Olive Oil
- Almonds
- Tilapia Fillet
- Tamari Soybean Sauce
- Worcestershire Sauce

- Canola Vegetable Oil
- Pork Chop with Center Loin and Bone In
- Cayenne Powder
- Yellow Mustard Seed
- Bone-in Chicken Wing

Phase 2 Meal Plan

Day One

(Total: Calories: 1252; fat: 71g; net carbs: 18.9g; protein: 79.1g)

Breakfast:

Fantastic Atkins Pie Crust (Calorie: 193; Fat: 13.6g: Carbohydrate: 2.5g; Protein: 14.8g)

Snack

Bony Chicken Wingettes (Calorie: 276; Fat: 18.5g: Carbohydrate: 3.4g; Protein: 22g)

Lunch

Flavorful Almond and Parmesan Crusted Tilapia (Calorie: 344; Fat: 21.9g: Carbohydrate: 6.6g; Protein: 29.3g)

Dinner

Dreamy Cali Mac and Cheese (Calorie: 320; Fat: 27g: Carbohydrate: 5.6g; Protein: 11.4g

Dessert

Chocolaty Chocolate Cream Frosty (Calorie: 119 ; Fat: 11.5g: Carbohydrate: 0.8g; Protein: 1.6g)

Day Two

(Totals: Calorie: 755; fat: 52.3g; net carbs: 24.6g; Protein: 76.9g)

Breakfast:

Delicious Almond and Coconut Muffin (Calorie: 405; Fat: 21; Carbohydrate: 3.5g; Dietary Fiber: 3g; Protein:9.7g)

Snack

Healthy Atkins Peanut Butter Granola Bar Parfait with Yogurt and Strawberries (Calorie: 314; Fat: 9.5g: Carbohydrate: 12.6g; Protein: 24.1g)

Lunch

Healthy Broiled Up Tilapia Parmesan (Calorie: 224; Fat: 12.8g: Carbohydrate: 0.8g; Protein: 25.4g)

Dinner

Tender Baked Tamari Lemon Pork Chops (Calorie: 149; Fat: 8g: Carbohydrate: 4g; Protein: 15.2g)

Dessert

Lightly Sweet Chocolate Brownie Drops (Calorie: 104; Fat: 9.4g: Carbohydrate: 3.9g; Protein: 2.5g)

Day Three

(Total: Calories: 1252; fat: 92.5g; net carbs: 18.9g; protein: 78.3g)

Breakfast:

Fantastic Atkins Pie Crust (Calorie: 193; Fat: 13.6g: Carbohydrate: 2.5g; Protein: 14.8g)

Snack

Bony Chicken Wingettes (Calorie: 276; Fat: 18.5g: Carbohydrate: 3.4g; Protein: 22g)

Lunch

Flavorful Almond and Parmesan Crusted Tilapia (Calorie: 344; Fat: 21.9g: Carbohydrate: 6.6g; Protein: 29.3g)

Dinner

Dreamy Cali Mac and Cheese (Calorie: 320; Fat: 27g: Carbohydrate: 5.6g; Protein: 11.4g

Dessert

Chocolaty Chocolate Cream Frosty (Calorie: 119 ; Fat: 11.5g: Carbohydrate: 0.8g; Protein: 1.6g)

Day Four

(Totals: Calorie: 1196; fat: 60.7g; net carbs: 24.8g; Protein: 77.1g)

Breakfast:

Delicious Almond and Coconut Muffin (Calorie: 405; Fat: 21; Carbohydrate: 3.5g; Dietary Fiber: 3g; Protein:9.7g)

Snack

Healthy Atkins Peanut Butter Granola Bar Parfait with Yogurt and Strawberries (Calorie: 314; Fat: 9.5g: Carbohydrate: 12.6g; Protein: 24.1g)

Lunch

Healthy Broiled Up Tilapia Parmesan (Calorie: 224; Fat: 12.8g: Carbohydrate: 0.8g; Protein: 25.4g)

Dinner

Tender Baked Tamari Lemon Pork Chops (Calorie: 149; Fat: 8g: Carbohydrate: 4g; Protein: 15.2g)

Dessert

Lightly Sweet Chocolate Brownie Drops (Calorie: 104; Fat: 9.4g: Carbohydrate: 3.9g; Protein: 2.5g)

Day Five

(Total: Calories: 1078; fat: 91.6g; net carbs: 18.9g; protein: 79.1g)

Breakfast:

Fantastic Atkins Pie Crust (Calorie: 193; Fat: 13.6g: Carbohydrate: 2.5g; Protein: 14.8g)

Snack

Bony Chicken Wingettes (Calorie: 276; Fat: 18.5g: Carbohydrate: 3.4g; Protein: 22g)

Lunch

Flavorful Almond and Parmesan Crusted Tilapia (Calorie: 344; Fat: 21.9g: Carbohydrate: 6.6g; Protein: 29.3g)

Dinner

Dreamy Cali Mac and Cheese (Calorie: 320; Fat: 27g: Carbohydrate: 5.6g; Protein: 11.4g

Dessert

Chocolaty Chocolate Cream Frosty (Calorie: 119 ; Fat: 11.5g: Carbohydrate: 0.8g; Protein: 1.6g)

Day Six

(Totals: Calorie: 1196; fat: 60.7g; net carbs: 24.8g; Protein: 76.9g)

Breakfast:

Delicious Almond and Coconut Muffin (Calorie: 405; Fat: 21; Carbohydrate: 3.5g; Dietary Fiber: 3g; Protein: 76.9g)

Snack

Healthy Atkins Peanut Butter Granola Bar Parfait with Yogurt and Strawberries (Calorie: 314; Fat: 9.5g: Carbohydrate: 12.6g; Protein: 24.1g)

Lunch

Healthy Broiled Up Tilapia Parmesan (Calorie: 224; Fat: 12.8g: Carbohydrate: 0.8g; Protein: 25.4g)

Dinner

Tender Baked Tamari Lemon Pork Chops (Calorie: 149; Fat: 8g: Carbohydrate: 4g; Protein: 15.2g)

Dessert

Lightly Sweet Chocolate Brownie Drops (Calorie: 104; Fat: 9.4g: Carbohydrate: 3.9g; Protein: 2.5g)

Day Seven

(Total: Calories: 1252; fat: 92.5g; net carbs: 18.9g; protein: 108.4g)

Breakfast:

Fantastic Atkins Pie Crust (Calorie: 193; Fat: 13.6g: Carbohydrate: 2.5g; Protein: 14.8g)

Snack

Bony Chicken Wingettes (Calorie: 276; Fat: 18.5g: Carbohydrate: 3.4g; Protein: 22g)

Lunch

Flavorful Almond and Parmesan Crusted Tilapia (Calorie: 344; Fat: 21.9g: Carbohydrate: 6.6g; Protein: 29.3g)

Dinner

Dreamy Cali Mac and Cheese (Calorie: 320; Fat: 27g: Carbohydrate: 5.6g; Protein: 11.4g)

Dessert

Chocolaty Chocolate Cream Frosty (Calorie: 119 ; Fat: 11.5g: Carbohydrate: 0.8g; Protein: 1.6g)

Once you have attained a weight that just 4.5kg away from your goal, you are ready to enter phase 3. Here, you are going to want to add even more carbs to your diet and keep following this until you slow down losing weight.

Phase 3 Shopping List

- Salt as required
- Sucralose based Sweetener
- Cinnamon
- Unsalted Butter Stick
- Low Carb Baking Mix
- Tap Water
- Almond Meal Flour
- High Fiber Coconut Flour (Organic)
- Cinnamon
- Baking Powder
- Egg
- Extra Virgin Olive Oil
- Butter filled boneless pork loin chops
- Blue Cheese

- Bacon slices
- Garlic
- Ground Pepper as required
- Fresh Parsley
- Parmesan Cheese
- Softened Butter
- Red Tomato
- Cilantro
- Red Onion
- Jalapeno Popper
- Avocado
- Mayonnaise
- Lemon Juice
- Basil
- Onion Powder
- Celery Salt
- Greek Yogurt
- Atkins Peanut Butter Granola Bar
- Large Strawberries
- Olive Oil
- Almonds
- Tilapia Fillet
- Tamari Soybean Sauce
- Worcestershire Sauce

- Canola Vegetable Oil
- Pork Chop with Center Loin and Bone In
- Cayenne Powder
- Yellow Mustard Seed
- Bone-in Chicken Wing

Phase 3 Meal Plan

Day One

(Total: Calories: 1112; fat: 296g; net carbs: 47.4g; protein: 75.6g)

Breakfast:

Fantastic Atkins Pie Crust (Calorie: 193; Fat: 13.6g: Carbohydrate: 2.5g; Protein: 14.8g)

Snack

Melty Apricot Apple Cloud (Calorie: 9.9; Fat: 22.4g: Carbohydrate: 25g; Protein: 1.5g)

Lunch

Over Simplified Barbeque Chicken (Calorie: 330; Fat: 14g: Carbohydrate: 2.6g; Protein: 45.6g)

Dinner

Dreamy Cali Mac and Cheese (Calorie: 320; Fat: 27g: Carbohydrate: 5.6g; Protein: 11.4g)

Dessert

Juicy Berries With Chocolate Ganache (Calorie: 260 ; Fat: 17.8g: Carbohydrate: 11.7g; Protein: 2.3g)

Day Two

(Total: Calories: 1130; fat: 80.1g; net carbs: 20.1; protein: 75.6g)

Breakfast:

Beautiful Apple Muffin With Cinnamon Pecan Streusel (Calorie: 242; Fat: 20.6g: Carbohydrate: 5.3g; Protein: 7.5g)

Snack

Bony Chicken Wingettes (Calorie: 276; Fat: 18.5g: Carbohydrate: 3.4g; Protein: 22g)

Lunch

Flavorful Almond and Parmesan Crusted Tilapia (Calorie: 344; Fat: 21.9g: Carbohydrate: 6.6g; Protein: 29.3g)

Dinner

Tender Baked Tamari Lemon Pork Chops (Calorie: 149; Fat: 8g: Carbohydrate: 4g; Protein: 15.2g)

Dessert

Chocolaty Cream Frosty (Calorie: 119 ; Fat: 11.1g: Carbohydrate: 0.8g; Protein: 1.6g)

Day Three

(Total: Calories: 1526; fat: 87.8g; net carbs: 27.9; protein: 125.9g)

Breakfast:

Fantastic Atkins Pie Crust (Calorie: 193; Fat: 13.6g: Carbohydrate: 2.5g; Protein: 14.8g)

Snack

Healthy Atkins Peanut Butter Granola Bar (Calorie: 314; Fat: 9.5g: Carbohydrate: 12.6g; Protein: 24.1g)

Lunch

Tasty Apricot Glazed Brisket (Calorie: 358; Fat: 16g: Carbohydrate: 1.3g; Protein: 47g)

Dinner

Tantalizing Cheddar Omelet With Avocado and Salsa (Calorie: 419; Fat: 33.6g: Carbohydrate: 5.2g; Protein: 20.8g)

Dessert

Colorful Blueberry Cloud Muffin (Calorie: 242 ; Fat: 15.1g: Carbohydrate: 6.3g; Protein: 19.2g)

Day Four

(Total: Calories: 1088; fat: 78.4g; net carbs: 21.2; protein: 72.7g)

Breakfast:

Delicious Almond and Coconut Muffin (Calorie: 207; Fat: 16.8g: Carbohydrate: 3.5g; Protein: 9.7g)

Snack

Bony Chicken Wingettes (Calorie: 276; Fat: 18.5g: Carbohydrate: 3.4g; Protein: 22g)

Lunch

Flavorful Almond and Parmesan Crusted Tilapia (Calorie: 344; Fat: 21.9g: Carbohydrate: 6.6g; Protein: 29.3g)

Dinner

A Pudding From Yorkshire (Calorie: 157; Fat: 11.8g: Carbohydrate: 3.8g; Protein: 9.2g)

Dessert

Lightly Sweet Chocolate Brownie Drops (Calorie: 104; Fat: 9.4g: Carbohydrate: 3.9g; Protein: 2.5g)

Day Five

(Total: Calories: 689; fat: 47.9g; net carbs: 25.1; protein: 44.8g)

Breakfast:

Fantastic Atkins Pie Crust (Calorie: 193; Fat: 13.6g: Carbohydrate: 2.5g; Protein: 14.8g)

Snack

Greenful Avocado Salsa (Calorie: 71; Fat: 5.3g: Carbohydrate: 3.3g; Protein: 1.1g)

Lunch

Health Broiled Up Tilapia Parmesan (Calorie: 224; Fat: 12.8g: Carbohydrate: 0.8; Protein: 24.5g)

Dinner

Spicy Red Bell Pepper Filled Up With Cherry Tomatoes And Feta (Calorie: 97; Fat: 6.8g: Carbohydrate: 4.6g; Protein: 1.9g)

Dessert

Lightly Sweet Chocolate Brownie Drops (Calorie: 104; Fat: 9.4g: Carbohydrate: 13.9g; Protein: 2.5g)

Day Six

(Total: Calories: 1301; fat: 94.2g; net carbs: 31.7; protein: 85g)

Breakfast:

Crunchy Protein Pancakes (Calorie: 101; Fat: 9.9g: Carbohydrate: 4.4g; Protein: 20g)

Snack

Bony Chicken Wingettes (Calorie: 276; Fat: 18.5g: Carbohydrate: 3.4g; Protein: 22g)

Lunch

Flavorful Almond and Parmesan Crusted Tilapia (Calorie: 344; Fat: 21.9g: Carbohydrate: 6.6g; Protein: 29.3g)

Dinner

Dreamy Cali Mac and Cheese (Calorie: 320; Fat: 27g: Carbohydrate: 5.6g; Protein: 11.4g)

Dessert

Juicy Berries With Chocolate Ganache (Calorie: 260 ; Fat: 17.8g: Carbohydrate: 11.7g; Protein: 2.3g)

Day Seven

(Total: Calories: 1443; fat: 108g; net carbs: 25.7g; protein: 81.9gg)

Breakfast:

Fantastic Atkins Pie Crust (Calorie: 193; Fat: 13.6g: Carbohydrate: 2.5g; Protein: 14.8g)

Snack

Bony Chicken Wingettes (Calorie: 276; Fat: 18.5g: Carbohydrate: 3.4g; Protein: 22g)

Lunch

Flavorful Almond and Parmesan Crusted Tilapia (Calorie: 344; Fat: 21.9g: Carbohydrate: 6.6g; Protein: 29.3g)

Dinner

Dreamy Cali Mac and Cheese (Calorie: 320; Fat: 27g: Carbohydrate: 5.6g; Protein: 11.4g)

Dessert

Fantastic Caramelized Custard (Calorie: 310 ; Fat: 27g: Carbohydrate: 7.6g; Protein: 4.4g)

Phase 4

Once you are done with phase 3 and have reached a level where you are about to gain weight. Move into the phase 4 where all you can choose your meals as you wish. Just keep a medium level carbohydrate intake, and you are set!

Chapter 3:
Mouth-watering Breakfast

Crunchy Almond Protein Pancakes

(Prepping time: 5 minutes\ Cooking time: 10 minutes |For 4 servings)

Start your day with a fine dish of protein filled pancakes with crunchy almonds sprinkled all over with a nice bite.

Ingredients:

- 2 ounce of Vanilla Whey Protein
- ¼ cup of Almond Meal Flour
- 3 tablespoon Whole Grain Soy Flour
- 1 teaspoon of Baking Powder
- 3 large sized whole eggs
- 1/3 cup of large creamed cottage cheese

Preparation:

1) Start off by taking a bowl and mixing up the almond meal, protein powder, baking powder and soy flour finely
2) Then whisk up your eggs and blend them with your cottage cheese
3) Mix up both the mixtures together to form the batter

4) On a lightly greased up (with butter) skillet placed over medium heat, pour about ¼ cup of Pancake batter for each pancake
5) Once bubble begins to form at the middle, turn it over and cook for about 2 minutes
6) Keep repeating the process until all batter are used up

Nutrition Values

- Calories: 191
- Fat: 9.9g
- Carbohydrates: 4.4g
- Protein: 20g
- Dietary Fiber: 1.6g

Delicious Almond and Coconut Muffin

(Prepping time: 3 minutes\ Cooking time: 1 minutes |For 1 servings)

We all love cupcakes right? Why not give a fine treat to yourself by crafting a beautiful cupcake topped up with nice bits of premium almond.

Ingredients:

- 2 tablespoon of Almond Meal Flour
- 1/3 tablespoon of Sucralose Based Sweetener
- 1/3 tablespoon of Organic High Fiber Coconut Flour
- ½ a teaspoon of Cinnamon
- ¼ teaspoon of Baking Powder
- 1/8 teaspoon of Salt
- 1 large sized Egg
- 1 teaspoon of Extra Virgin Olive Oil

Preparation:

1) For this relatively simple recipe, you are first going to want to take a coffee mug and toss in all of the dry ingredients in it
2) Next, toss in the egg and pour oil and keep stirring it until nicely combined
3) Microwave the mixture for about 1 minute, after which it should be prepared. Just used a knife to cut it out and serve with butter and eat

Nutrition Values

- Calories: 207
- Fat: 16.8g
- Carbohydrates: 3.5g
- Protein: 9.7g
- Dietary Fiber: 3g

Smooth Almond Pineapple Smoothie

(Prepping time: 5 minutes\ Cooking time: 1 minutes |For 1 servings)

Sometimes it is essential to go for something a bit chilly no? This pineapple smoothie will chill your internals after a long night work and keep you energetic for the rest of the day.

Ingredients:

- ½ cup of Plain Yoghurt
- 2 and a ½ ounce of Pineapple
- 20 whole pieces of Blanched & Silvered Almonds
- ½ a cup of Pure Almond Milk

Preparation:

1) Take a blender and mix up all of the ingredients listed and finely puree it until it is nicely creamy and smooth
2) Chill it up further more if you want, and sip it up as to freshen yourself up

Nutrition Values

- Calories: 280
- Fat: 18.6g
- Carbohydrates: 17g
- Protein: 10.8g
- Dietary Fiber: 4.2g

Beautiful Apple Muffin With Cinnamon-Pecan Streusel

(Prepping time: 15 minutes\ Cooking time: 25 minutes |For 8 servings)

While you may not be a big fan of Cinnamon, these apple muffins will definitely bring back your love of cinnamon once again!

Ingredients:

- 1 and a 2/3 cup of Almond Meal Flour
- ½ a cup of half Pecans
- 6 and a ½ teaspoon of Cinnamon
- 1/3 teaspoon of salt
- 24 teaspoon of Erythritol
- 1 pinch of Stevia
- 2 tablespoon of Unsalted Butter Stick
- 2 large sized Whole Egg
- ¼ cup of coconut Unsweetened Butter Stick
- 2 teaspoon of Vanilla Extract
- 2 tablespoon of Organic high Fiber Coconut flour

- 1 teaspoon of Baking Powder
- 2/3 cup of quartered or chopped Apples

Preparation:

1) The first step here is to pre-heat your oven to a temperature of 350 degree Fahrenheit
2) Take a muffin tin and prepare it with about 8 cupcake papers
3) Take a small bowl and mix up your 2/3 cup of almond flour, chopped up pecans, 2 tablespoon of your cinnamon, 2 tablespoon of granular sugar substitute, 1/8 teaspoon of your salt, just a pinch of stevia and mix in about 2 tablespoon of melted butter
4) Mix everything using a fork and gently create the batter
5) As for the muffins, all you have to take another bowl and whisk in the eggs, 2 teaspoon of vanilla, ¼ cup of coconut milk, just a pinch of stevia, about 6 tablespoon of granular sugar substitute, about ½ teaspoon of the ground cinnamon .

6) Then, add in just a cup of almond flour followed by 2 tablespoon of coconut flour, 1 teaspoon baking powder, ¼ teaspoon of salt and mix everything together only to fold in with some finely chopped up apples
7) Divide the whole mixture into your muffin tin (8 portions) and top each of them off with 2 tablespoon of streusel
8) Let it bake for about 25 minutes and remove it too cool for 20 minutes
9) Serve
10)   Keep in mind that it is possible to store them in airtight containers for about a week

Nutrition Values

- Calories: 242
- Fat: 20.6g
- Carbohydrates: 5.3g
- Protein: 7.5g
- Dietary Fiber: 4.2g

Fantastic Atkins Cinnamon Pie Crust

(Prepping time: 10 minutes\ Cooking time: 30 minutes |For 8 servings)

This is a fantastic Pie Crust base which you can use to make all sorts of Pie! No more will you need to wait for buying up a Atkins compatible Pie Crust. It's all at your home.

Ingredients:

- ¼ teaspoon of Salt
- 1 teaspoon of Sucralose based Sweetener
- 1 teaspoon of Cinnamon
- ½ cup of unsalted butter stick
- 3 pieces of ¾ serving of all purpose low-carb baking mix
- 2 tablespoon of tap water

Preparation:

1) The first step is to take food processor and pulse up the baking mix, cinnamon, sugar substitute properly

and mix them up for about 30 seconds until a coarse meal is formed

2) Pulse in a little bit of water to make sure that the dough is perfectly mixed up and pulse for more 30 seconds

3) Once the dough it ready, transfer it to a sheet of plastic wrap and finely form it into disk of 3 inch radius.

4) Wrap it up very tightly and freeze them for about 30 minutes

5) Roll it up and bake it to make a nice cruse for your pie

Nutrition Values

- Calories: 193
- Fat: 13.6g
- Carbohydrates: 2.5g
- Protein: 14.8g
- Dietary Fiber: 1.7g

Buttery Soft Cuisine Waffles

(Prepping time: 10 minutes\ Cooking time: 30 minutes |For 8 servings)

This is a very premium level and soft cuisine waffle. Top it with a good amount of honey to give a sweet treat to your morning sweet tooth!

Ingredients:

- 1 packet of Sucralose Based Sweetener
- 1 large sized whole egg
- 2 teaspoon of baking powder
- ¼ teaspoon of salt
- 1 cup of half and half cream
- 3 serving of all purpose low carb baking mix

Preparation:

1) Take large sized bowl and toss in the baking mix, sugar, baking powder, sugar substitute alongside just an amount of salt
2) Take another large sized bowl and mix up the cream and the egg

3) Toss in the dry ingredients and mix it up nicely and keep beating it until no lumps are there
4) Let the whole mix sit for about 5 minutes for the baking powder to be activated
5) Take you waffle iron and heat it up nicely. Then pour in the batter in the center of iron
6) Close it up and let it cook for about 11 and a ½ minute until a golden brown texture has been achieved
7) Keep repeating it until the whole mixture is used

Nutrition Values

- Calories: 193
- Fat: 9g
- Carbohydrates: 5.9g
- Protein: 21.4g
- Dietary Fiber: 1.9g

Sweet Bell Pepper Rings Filled Up With Egg and Mozzarella With Fruit

(Prepping time: 10 minutes\ Cooking time: 5 minutes |For 1 servings)

Bell peppers are usually spicy! With this recipe you will be able to prepare bell peppers that blend a slight flavor of mozzarella cheese and eggy sweetness.

Ingredients:

- ¼ cup of shredded up whole Mozzarella Cheese Milk
- 1 teaspoon of Extra Virgin Olive Oil
- ¼ small sized bananas
- ¼ pieces of small Apples
- ½ a fruit of Kiwi
- 2 large sized whole egg
- ¼ cup of raspberries
- ½ of a medium sized sweet red pepper

Preparation:

1) The first step here is to cut up the bell pepper into piece of 1 inch rounds
2) Then you are to take a nice skillet and heat it up with just a small amount of oil over medium level of heat
3) Into each of your round, crack in the egg and cook it for about 2 minutes
4) Pour in about 1-2 tablespoon of water
5) Steam the eggs and pepper for about 3-5 minutes until the eggs are finely cooked
6) Top them up finally with some cheese and cover it up for about a minute to allow the cheese to melt
7) Finally, combine up the fruits and serve nicely with the pepper rounds

Nutrition Values

- Calories: 361
- Fat: 20g
- Carbohydrates: 20.1g
- Protein: 19.9g
- Dietary Fiber: 5.8g

Finely Baked Egg and Asparagus
(Prepping time: 5 minutes \ Cooking time: 10 minutes |For 1 servings)

Sometimes we just need to go for something on the lighter side of the spectrum! Bake up a finely prepared omelet for the whole family and encourage them to follow you into an Atkins Diet.

Ingredients:

- 8 small spear of 5 inch Asparagus
- ¼ cup of heavy cream
- 2 whole sized large eggs
- 2 tablespoon of Almond Meal Flour
- 1 tablespoon of Parmesan Cheese
- 1/8 teaspoon of garlic
- 1/8 teaspoon of Black Pepper

Preparation:

1) The first step is to pre-heat your 400 degree Fahrenheit
2) Take a small sized oven safe casserole and grease it up with oil

3) Boil up your asparaguses for about 2 minutes until nicely tender
4) Drain them up and run them under cold water and pat them dry
5) Finely arrange everything in a baking dish
6) Take your cream and pour them over your asparagus and finely crack your eggs on top of them
7) Take a small sized bowl and blend up your almond meal, garlic, black pepper and parmesan cheese together
8) Sprinkle everything on top of your eggs
9) Cook the egg for about 5-10 minutes and final, take it out once the cream has puffed over the edges and serve it hot

Nutrition Values

- Calories: 471
- Fat: 40g
- Carbohydrates: 5.6g
- Protein: 20.8g
- Dietary Fiber: 4g

Chapter 4: Delicious Lunch

Healthy Broiled Up Tilapia Parmesan

(Prepping time: 5 minutes\ Cooking time: 10 minutes |For 8 servings)

Fishes are in general regarded as pretty healthy edibles. But that doesn't necessarily mean that they are always as delicious! However, you can change that up using just a bit of Parmesan cheese and this recipe.

Ingredients:

- ½ a cup of Parmesan Cheese
- ¼ cup of softened butter
- 3 tablespoon of mayonnaise
- 2 tablespoon of fresh lemon juice
- ¼ teaspoon of dried basil
- ¼ teaspoon of ground black pepper
- 1/8 teaspoon of onion powder
- 1/8 teaspoon of celery salt
- 2 pound of tilapia fillet

Preparation:

1) This recipe can be prepared in just 2 very simple and easy to follow steps. The first one is to take a broiling pan and pan it nicely with aluminum foil
2) Take another small sized bowl and mix everything up together (Parmesan, mayo, butter, lemon juice)
3) Season it nicely with dried up basil, onion powder, pepper, and of course the celery salt
4) Finally, arrange your fillets in a nice singular layer on your pan and broil a few inches from the heat for about 2 minutes
5) Flip them over and broil for a more few minutes
6) Remove the fillets from your pan and cover the upper layer with your parmesan cheese mixture
7) Broil for another 2 minutes making sure that the toppings are browned
8) Serve

Nutrition Values

- Calories: 224
- Fat: 12.8g
- Carbohydrates: 0.8g
- Protein: 25.4g
- Dietary Fiber: 0.1g

Healthy Blue Cheese, Bacon and Chive Stuffed Up Pork Chops

(Prepping time: 15 minutes\ Cooking time: 20 minutes |For 2 servings)

This recipe will allow you to combine a number of different ingredients including blue cheese and chive tossed in with bacon to create a powerful bash of multitude flavors.

Ingredients:

- 2 pieces of butter flied boneless pork loin chops
- 4 ounces of crumbled up blue cheese
- 2 slices of cooked and crumbled up bacon
- 2 tablespoon of freshly chopped up chives
- Garlic as needed
- Ground black pepper as needed
- Chopped up fresh parsley just for the garnish

Preparation:

1) The first step here is to pre-heat your oven to a temperature of 325 degree Fahrenheit
2) Take a shallow baking dish and grease it up with butter
3) Take a small sized bowl and mix in the blue cheese, chive and bacon
4) Dive it into two halves and pack them up in a loosely shaped ball
5) Place the ball in the pocket of your butterflied pork chop and close it up only to secure it using tooth picks
6) Season the chops with garlic, pepper and salt
7) Bake for about 20 minutes inside your pre-heated oven until the stuffing is finely
8) Lastly, garnish it up with some parsley and swallow up

Nutrition Values

- Calories: 394
- Fat: 26.3g
- Carbohydrates: 2g
- Protein: 36g
- Dietary Fiber: 0.3g

Succulent Pan Fried Tuna Patty

(Prepping time: 15 minutes\ Cooking time: 5 minutes |For 2 servings)

Everybody loves Tuna! But you know what else we love? Burger patties! Go ahead with this recipe prepare you juicy tuna patties to create your own Atkins diet burger.

Ingredients:

- 1 can of tuna packed in water that has to be drained out later on
- 1 piece of whole egg
- ½ a stalk of chopped up celery
- 2 tablespoon of mayonnaise
- 2 tablespoon of chopped up walnut
- 2 tablespoon of freshly chopped parsley
- 1 teaspoon of chopped up fresh dill
- 1 tablespoon of butter
- ¼ up of shredded Cheddar Cheese

Preparation:

1) The first step here is to take bowl and stir in your tuna, egg, mayonnaise, parsley,

celery, walnuts and ill only to mix them up properly until they are combined

2) Using the mixture, form two pieces of fine patty
3) Take your skillet and melt butter over medium heat and cook the patties in the molten butter until a nice golden texture has appeared for about 2-3 minutes
4) Flip the patty and top it up with cheddar cheese
5) Keep cooking until the other side is golden brown as well
6) Done

Nutrition Values

- Calories: 367
- Fat: 29.3g
- Carbohydrates: 2.4g
- Protein: 24.2g
- Dietary Fiber: 0.8g

Luscious Crust less Quiche Lori-Iane

(Prepping time: 10 minutes\ Cooking time: 210 minutes |For 8 servings)

Even though this recipe has a weird name, it still goes to a great extent to simulate the flavor of a pizza with its combination of feta and parmesan packed with a healthy dose of vegetable goodness.

Ingredients:

- 4 pieces of eggs
- 16 ounce container of sour cream
- 10 ounce of packaged up frozen and chopped up spinach
- 1 cup of shredded up cheese
- ½ a cup of crumbled up feta cheese
- ½ a cup of shredded up parmesan cheese
- ½ a cup of chopped up onion
- ½ a cup of chopped up tomato

- 4 ounce of chopped up green chiles all drained up
- 1 minced up teaspoon of garlic
- 1 teaspoon of chopped up ground cumin
- 1 tablespoon of paprika
- ¼ teaspoon of cayenne pepper

Preparation:

1) The first step is to pre-heat your oven to a temperature of 325 degree Fahrenheit
2) The next step is to beat up your eggs in a bowl and whisk in the sour cream and keep mixing it until finely smoothened
3) After that, mix in your spinach alongside the cheddar cheese, parmesan cheese, feta cheese, tomato, onion, green chiles, cumin, garlic, cayenne pepper and paprika
4) Take a plate and pour in the egg mixture into that pie plate
5) Set up your pie plate on a prepared baking sheet and keep baking the quiche until about 1 hour

Nutrition Values

- Calories: 401
- Fat: 32.4g
- Carbohydrates: 10.6g
- Protein: 19.3g
- Dietary Fiber: 2.5g

Asian Beef Salad

(Prepping time: 720 minutes\ Cooking time: 5 minutes |For 1 servings)

Just because Atkins diet requires us to go for green vegetables, doesn't mean that that's the only thing we can eat! The Asian beef salad is perfect for those who are looking to penetrate into the world of Atkins diet but are still not quite ready to let go of meat.

Ingredients:

- ½ a clove of garlic
- ½ a tablespoon of Tamari Soybean Sauce
- ¼ tablespoon of Sodium And Sugar Free Rice Vinegar
- ¼ teaspoon of Sesame Oil
- 1/8 teaspoon of Based Sweetener
- 1/8 teaspoon of Curry powder
- 1/16 teaspoon of ginger
- 4 pieces of ¼ ounce Beef Top Sirloin
- ¾ cup of spring mix salad

- ½ a tablespoon of Canola Vegetable Oil
- ¼ of large sized sweet Red Pepper
- 2 ounce of Waterchest nuts
- 1 large sized Scallion

Preparation:

1) The first step here is to take a bowl and mix in the green onion, rice wine vinegar, soy sauce, sesame oil, sugar and mix them well.
2) Take a resalable bag and put the steak in the it alongside half of the mixture, and let it marinate over night
3) For the remaining soy sauce mixture, toss in the curry powder alongside the ginger.
4) Take a nice skillet and heat it up alongside the canola oil over high heat until it is very hot
5) Bring out the beef from the fridge and drain and discard the marinade
6) Quickly stir fry it on your heated skillet and transfer it to a large bowl

7) Toss in the salad greens, water chest nuts, bell pepper alongside the soy sauce and cover up your beef with the mixture only to serve hot and immediately

Nutrition Values

- Calories: 295
- Fat: 13.3g
- Carbohydrates: 10.4g
- Protein: 29.5g
- Dietary Fiber: 4.1g

Flavorful Almond And Parmesan Crusted Tilapia

(Prepping time: 10 minutes\ Cooking time: 1-minutes |For 4 servings)

Yet another recipe involving tilapia. But this time, it is more much more crunchier in nature thanks to the addition of Almond.

Ingredients:

- 1 teaspoon of olive oil
- 3 minced cloves of garlic
- ½ a cup of grated parmesan
- ¼ cup of buttery spread
- ¼ cup of crushed silvered almonds
- 3 tablespoon of reduced fat olive oil mayonnaise
- 2 tablespoon of bread crumb
- 2 tablespoon of fresh lemon juice
- 1 teaspoon of seafood seasoning
- ¼ teaspoon of dried basil
- ¼ teaspoon of ground black pepper
- 1/8 teaspoon of celery salt

- 1 pound of tilapia fillets

Preparation:

1) The first step here is to set up your oven rack about 6 inches from the heat source of your oven and pre-heat your oven's broiler portion
2) Line up your broiling pan with a cooking spray
3) Take a skillet over medium level heat and pour in some olive oil to heat it up and toss your garlic to cook them until a nice fragrance is out. This should take no more than 5 minutes
4) Take a bowl and mix up the parmesan, buttery spread, garlic, mayonnaise, almonds, lemon juice, mayonnaise, bread crumbs, seasoning, seafood, onion powder, basil, black pepper and lastly celery salt
5) IN your prepared pan, lay your tilapia fillets in fine single layered section and cover it up with aluminum foil

6) Broil up in your pre-heated oven for about 3 minutes then flip up the fillets cover it again with your foil and broil once again for 3 minutes
7) Remove the foil and pour in the cheese mix
8) Broil yet again until the top of the fish is browned which should take no more than 2 minutes
9) Serve hot

Nutrition Values

- Calories: 344
- Fat: 21.9g
- Carbohydrates: 6.6g
- Protein: 29.3g
- Dietary Fiber: 0.9g

Tasty Apricot Glazed Brisket

(Prepping time: 15 minutes\ Cooking time: 5 minutes |For 2 servings)

When it comes to Briskets, people always have multiple opinions. But with this finely glazed Apricot Brisket! You will have no trouble winning the heart of everyone out there.

Ingredients:

- 4 pound of beef brisket
- 2 teaspoon of salt
- 2 teaspoon of paprika
- 1 teaspoon of Black Pepper
- 3 tablespoon of Sugar Free Apricot

Preparation:

1) The first step here is to pre-heat your oven to a temperature of 475 degree Fahrenheit

2) Season them up with salt and brisket alongside pepper and paprika
3) Gently place your brisket on your Dutch oven with the brisket fat side facing down
4) Scatter the carrots and onions around the beef nicely and let it cook for 15 minutes
5) Once done, turn over the brisket with the fat side up and add just about ½ a cup of water to cover it tightly
6) Drop down the temperature to 375 degree Fahrenheit and let it cook for about 3-4 hours until the brisket is finely tender
7) Heat up your broiler and remove the brisket from your oven and place it on the broiler pan finely
8) Spread jam all over your brisket and broil 6 from heat sources for about 5 minutes until the jam has light brown spots
9) While the brisket is being broiled, gently remove the onion and carrots from the cooking juice
10) Cover up your brisket with foil and let it rest for the next 15 minutes

11) Gently remove the surface fat and finely serve it with the degreased cooking juices

Nutrition Values

- Calories: 358
- Fat: 16g
- Carbohydrates: 1.3g
- Protein: 47g
- Dietary Fiber: 0.3g

Over Simplified Barbeque Chicken

(Prepping time: 10 minutes\ Cooking time: 90 minutes |For 6 servings)

Making BBQ chicken on the go might be a hassle as it requires quite a few steps to go through. This recipe is designed to make the process of BBQ-ing your chickens as easy as possible without sacrificing on the taste.

Ingredients:

- 6 bone-in chicken breast halves skin on
- 1 tablespoon of Worcestershire sauce
- 1 tablespoon of hickory flavored liquid smoke
- 2 teaspoon of chili powder
- 2 teaspoon of ground cumin
- 2 teaspoon garlic powder
- 2 teaspoon of dried thyme
- 2 teaspoon dried oregano
- Salt as needed
- Pepper as needed

Preparation:

1) The first step here is to pre-heat your oven to a temperature of 375 degree Fahrenheit
2) Then take a lightly greased up 9 inch by 13 inch baking dish and place the chicken pieces in a layer. Making sure to keep some space in between
3) Drizzle them up with the Worcestershire sauce, liquid smoke and the sprinkle some cumin, chili powder, garlic powder, oregano, thyme, pepper and salt
4) Cover up your dish with aluminum foil and bake it for about 1 and half hour
5) Serve

Nutrition Values

- Calories: 330
- Fat: 14g
- Carbohydrates: 2.6g
- Protein: 45.4g
- Dietary Fiber: 0.9g

Chapter 5: Graceful Snacks

Melty Apricot-Apple Cloud

(Prepping time: 65 minutes\ Cooking time: 10 minutes |For 6 servings)

Don't be alarmed by the name "Baby" here in this recipe. Even though the Apricot Apple Cloud might be targeted towards baby, you can also get a good punch out of this for your Atkins Snack time.

Ingredients:

- 1 and ½ cup of heavy cream
- 16 ounce of Baby Food Applesauce
- 2 tablespoon of Sucralose Based Sweetener

Preparation:

1) The firsts step here is to take an electric mixer and beat up your cream and sugar substitute properly until a nice firm peak is formed

2) Once it is done, gently fold in your food in nice jars
3) Divide the complete mixture amongst 6 deserts and let it chill for about an hour before serving it up

Nutrition Values

- Calories: 9.9
- Fat: 22.4
- Carbohydrates: 25g
- Protein: 1.5g
- Dietary Fiber: 1.1g

Magnificent Artichoke With Three Cheese

(Prepping time: 20 minutes\ Cooking time: 40 minutes |For 4 servings)

Yet another intelligent way to gobble up your green veggies by creating an amalgam of green veggies and three different kinds of cheeses! Yum.

Ingredients:

- 9 ounce of Artichoke
- ½ a cup of Bouillon vegetable broth
- 3 tablespoon of extra virgin olive oil
- 3 teaspoon of garlic
- 2 tablespoon of parsley
- 1 teaspoon of Fresh Lemon Juice
- ½ a cup of shredded Fontana Cheese
- 6 pieces of Basil Leaves
- ½ a cup of shredded Swiss cheese
- ½ a cup of Parmesan Cheese

Preparation:

1) The first step here is to pre-heat your oven to 400 degree Fahrenheit
2) Next, you are to arrange your artichokes I a fine single layer at the bottom of a 2 quart baking dish
3) Then nicely top it up with garlic and the broth
4) Drizzle it on top with a good amount of lemon juice and olive oil
5) Sprinkle in some basil and parsley as required
6) Cover the whole dish evenly with the different kind of cheeses, making sure that you end with Parmesan
7) Cover it up with the Aluminum Foil and bake it up until the artichoke has been fully tender. It should not take more than 15 minute for the cheese to melt
8) Once done, uncover the foil and finely bake until the cheese has been lightly golden colored and crusted . It should take more 25 minutes
9) Once done, remove it from the oven and let it cool only to serve to be eaten

Nutrition Values

- Calories: 57
- Fat: 14g
- Carbohydrates: 3g
- Protein: 4g
- Dietary Fiber: 2.6g

Healthy Atkins Peanut Butter Granola Bar Parfait with Strawberries And Yogurt

(Prepping time: 5 minutes\ Cooking time: 0 minutes |For 1 servings)

There is a misconception that Granola Bars are primarily targeted towards sports man and athletes. Well that is actually wrong! Granola Bars are excellent sources of energy and combined with yogurt and Strawberries, they can turn into great Atkins suitable Snack.

Ingredients:

- ½ a cup of Plain Greek Yoghurt
- 1 serving of Atkins Peanut Butter Granola Bar
- 5 large sized strawberries

Preparation:

1) The process is very easy. All you need to do is take a parfait glass and layer up the

chopped up granola bar alongside the yogurt and strawberries.

2) Chill it for a while if you want and serve

Nutrition Values

- Calories: 314
- Fat: 9.5g
- Carbohydrates: 12.6g
- Protein: 24.1g
- Dietary Fiber: 6.8g

Berryful Black Berry Peach Compote

(Prepping time: 10 minutes \ Cooking time: 20 minutes | For 12 servings)

An interesting meal originating from medieval Europe! This can be considered as both a snack and a desert and is a combination of cooked fruits, sugar and spices. If you are looking for something unique to add to your Atkins diet, go for this one! You won't regret it.

Ingredients:

- 4 ounce Sauvignon Blanc Wine
- 2 tablespoon of Xylitol
- 1 teaspoon of Ginger
- 1 teaspoon of Cinnamon
- 3 medium peaches
- 6 ounce blackberries
- ½ teaspoon Thick it Up

Preparation:

1) The first step here is to take a sauce pan and combine the wine, Xylitol, ginger, peaches and ground cinnamon
2) Then gently bring the mixture to a boil in a medium sized sauce pan and finely reduce the heat to a low level only to simmer it for 15 minutes
3) Toss in the black berries to that mixture until tender
4) Pour in the thick it Up and keep simmering for another 5 minutes
5) Remove the heat and let it cool to bring it down to room temperature

Nutrition Values

- Calories: 35
- Fat: 0.2g
- Carbohydrates: 4.2g
- Protein: 0.5g
- Dietary Fiber: 3.4g

Dried Tomatoes and Pine Nuts With Baked Brie

(Prepping time: 5 minutes\ Cooking time: 0 minutes |For 1 servings)

This is an amazing alternative to something reminiscent to a pancake or pudding, but much more healthier and packed with the juicy bites of tomatoes mixed with crunchy pine nuts.

Ingredients:

- ¼ cup of Frozen Black berries
- 1 cup of unsweetened coconut milk
- ¼ teaspoon of cinnamon
- ½ teaspoon of Vanilla extract
- 1 scoop of vanilla whey protein
- 1/16 teaspoon of Allspice Ground
- 1/16 cup of organic 100% whole ground golden flaxseed meal

Preparation:

1) For this recipe you are simply going to require to take a blender and take your unsweetened coconut milk and pour it in.
2) Later on, toss in your frozen blackberries, vanilla, protein powder, spice, milk and finely blender them up until smooth and nice texture has been achieved
3) Sip it up cold

Nutrition Values

- Calories: 221
- Fat: 9.8g
- Carbohydrates: 6.7g
- Protein: 21.8g
- Dietary Fiber: 5.8g

Indian Chicken Curry

(Prepping time: 8 minutes\ Cooking time: 20 minutes |For 6 servings)

Hailing from the mysterious continents of India, this curry is designed to give you the flavor of core Indian curries, while not going through the burden of collecting a myriad of spices! Imagine this as an Indian teaser!

Ingredients:

- 3 tablespoon of Unsalted Butter Stick
- 32 ounce of boneless chicken breast
- 1 teaspoon of cumin
- ½ a teaspoon of Coriander Leaf
- ½ a teaspoon of Ginger
- ¼ teaspoon of Crushed Red Pepper Flakes
- 2 teaspoon of Garlic
- ½ a cup of Chicken broth
- 1/3 cup of heavy cream
- 1/16 cup cilantro

Preparation:

1) The first step is to take a heavy skillet and put it over medium high level heat
2) Toss in your butter and let it foam around the butter sides
3) Toss in the chicken strips and cook it until finely browned, making sure to cook for 5 minutes every batch
4) Toss in the cumin, ginger, coriander, red-pepper flakes alongside the garlic and cook for 2 minutes stirring it continuously
5) Add in the chicken stock then and boil it up
6) Bring down the heat to medium-low level and simmer it for 5 minutes
7) Pour in the heavy cream then and simmer for another 3 minutes
8) Transfer the cooked chicken and gently serve it in a plate garnishing it with cilantro

Nutrition Values

- Calories: 413
- Fat: 22.1g
- Carbohydrates: 1g
- Protein: 49.1g
- Dietary Fiber: 0.3g

Greenful Avocado Salsa

(Prepping time: 10 minutes\ Cooking time: 0 minutes |For 4 servings)

Avocados are really great in general, but you can make it even more fantastic and green by chocking it up with a number of different vegetables to be a scoopful of green goodness.

Ingredients:

- 1 small sized whole Red tomato
- 1/8 cup of Cilantro
- 1 small sized Red Onion
- ½ of a Jalapeno Popper
- 1 piece of California Avocado
- 2 tablespoon of Fresh Lime Juice
- 1/8 teaspoon of Salt
- 1/8 teaspoon of Black pepper

Preparation:

1) The first step is to chop up your tomato alongside your cilantro and at the same

time, finely dice up your jalapeno and onion

2) Gently remove the outer skin off your avocado and chop It up only to place it on top of a nice serving bowl

3) Toss in the jalapeno, onion and also juice to the avocado mixture and combine finely.

4) Fold in the tomato along side the previously chopped up cilantro and season the whole mix with pepper and salt

5) Refrigerate it and serve!

Nutrition Values

- Calories: 71
- Fat: 5.3g
- Carbohydrates: 3.3g
- Protein: 1.1g
- Dietary Fiber: 3g

Bony Chicken Wingettes

(Prepping time: 10 minutes\ Cooking time: 35 minutes |For 8 servings)

Being an avid followed of Atkins might sometimes influence you to go ahead and try out a bucket of KFC chicken! Don't frown now, as this will get you just as close to that juicy goodness.

Ingredients:

- 2 tablespoon of Chili Powder
- 1 teaspoon of Cayenne Pepper
- 2 teaspoon of Yellow Mustard Seed
- 2 teaspoon of Salt
- ½ serving of All Purpose Low carb baking Mix
- 32 ounce of bone-in chicken wing

Preparation:

1) The first step here is to heat up your oven to a temperature of 450F

2) Take a jelly roll pan and line it up with foil and finely spray with cooking spray
3) Take a resalable bag and toss in your chili powder, cayenne mustard, 2 tablespoon of baking mix alongside salt to create your marinade
4) Then toss in half of your chicken wings and shake finely to coat them
5) Transfer them to the previously prepared pan and cook for about 30-35 minutes
6) Once done, serve in a platter

Nutrition Values

- Calories: 276
- Fat: 18.5g
- Carbohydrates: 3.4g
- Protein: 22.4g
- Dietary Fiber: 0.3g

Chapter 6:
Flavored
Desert

Colorful Blueberry Cloud Muffin

(Prepping time: 1 minutes\ Cooking time: 1 minutes |For 1 servings)

Famished after a whole day of work? Want to end the day on a sweet note? This colorful blueberry cloud muffin is the only thing you are going to need to lavish yourself into a goodnight sleep.

Ingredients:

- 1 ounce of Cream Cheese
- 1 large sized whole egg
- 2 tablespoon of Vanilla Whey Protein
- ¼ teaspoon of Baking Powder
- 1/8 teaspoon of Nutmeg
- ¼ cup of Blueberries

Preparation:

1) The first step here is to microwave your cream cheese in a mug for about 10-15 seconds
2) Toss in the egg and whisk it up alongside your cream cheese

3) Pour in the whey powder, nutmeg and baking powder only to mix them up properly
4) Toss in the blueberries them and mix yet again
5) Microwave for more 10-20 seconds
6) Run a knife from around the mug and take the cupcake out

Nutrition Values

- Calories: 242
- Fat: 15.1g
- Carbohydrates: 6.3g
- Protein: 19.2g
- Dietary Fiber: 0.9g

Classical Apple Tart

(Prepping time: 30 minutes\ Cooking time: 45 minutes |For 8 servings)

While there are hundreds of different apple tart recipes, nothing gets close to the original classic one! This Tart is all you are going to need to relive the past while being able to enjoy your Atkins routine properly.

Ingredients:

- 5 medium sized Apples
- ¼ cup of Sucralose Based Sweetener
- ¾ teaspoon of Cinnamon
- 1/8 Nutmeg
- 1 servings of Atkins Cuisine Pie Crust
- 1 tablespoon of Unsalted Butter Stick

Preparation:

1) I have already included a Atkins Pie Crust recipe, please follow that first to create the crust
2) Once done, heat up your oven to a temperature of 350 degree Fahrenheit

3) Take a large sized bowl and toss in the apples, cinnamon, nutmeg and sugar substitute
4) Make sure that the apples are finely coated all over
5) Then spoon the mixture into your crust and top it up with butter
6) Bake the tart for about 30 minutes
7) Cover it gent with a foil and bake for about 20 minutes until the apples are finely tenderized
8) Cool the tart on your cooling rack
9) Serve hot with a nice side of praline sauce and ice cream if you require

Nutrition Values

- Calories: 238
- Fat: 14.3g
- Carbohydrates: 18.1g
- Protein: 8.2g
- Dietary Fiber: 3.1g

Juicy Berries With Chocolate Ganache

(Prepping time: 10 minutes\ Cooking time: 5 minutes |For 6 servings)

You were waiting for a chocolate recipe weren't you? Well, this recipe will fulfill all of your chocolaty dreams with a carefully crafted chocolate Ganache dash with different kinds of berries to make it both healthy and mouthwatering for a chocolate buff.

Ingredients:

- 8 ounce of Strawberries
- 2 cups of Red Raspberries
- 2 cups of Fresh Blueberries
- 8 ounce of Sugar Free Chocolate Chips
- 1/3 cup of heavy cream
- ½ a teaspoon of Vanilla Extract

Preparation:

10)   Take about 6 desert bowls and toss in the fruits and combine them nicely

11) Take a saucepan and put it over slightly low heat
12)   Toss in the chocolate and cream only to melt them
13)   Then pour in the vanilla and keep stirring them until nicely smoothened
14)   Let it cool and drizzle a good amount of sauce over your fruits to serve

Nutrition Values

- Calories: 260
- Fat: 17.8g
- Carbohydrates: 11.7g
- Protein: 2.3g
- Dietary Fiber: 7.4g

Fantastic Caramelized Pear Custard

(Prepping time: 10 minutes\ Cooking time: 20 minutes |For 8 servings)

You might love pear, but that doesn't mean you might be willing to go for it all the time! But after caramelizing them with butter, you won't be able to stop yourself from swallowing them up!

Ingredients:

- 2 tablespoon of Butter
- 2 tablespoon of Xylitol
- ¼ teaspoon of Ground Cardamom
- 2 medium sized Pears
- 3 large sized whole egg
- 2 large sized egg yolks
- 2 cups of heavy cream
- 18 cup of sugar free low calorie maple flavor syrup
- ½ FL ounce of Rum

- 1 teaspoon of vanilla extract

Preparation:

1) Start this off by pre-heating your oven to a temperature of 375 degree Fahrenheit
2) The next step here is to take a large sauce pan and put it over medium-high level heat and toss in your xylitol, butter and cardamom
3) Once the butter has shown a molten texture toss in your pears only to allow it to caramelize. Make sure to give 4 minutes to each side
4) Gently remove the heat and arrange the whole in a pie plate
5) Store about 2 tablespoon of the syrup and pour the remaining on top of your pears
6) Take a small sized bowl and whisk up your egg yolks, eggs sugar free syrup, heavy cream, vanilla and run to mix them thoroughly
7) Then gently pour in the mixture over your pears and bake it for about 15-20 minutes until a golden brown texture has

appeared and the custard has set in nicely

8) Gently remove it from the oven and let it cool

9) Take a pastry brush and finely brush the top of your pear with the reserved syrup

10)   Serve

Nutrition Values

- Calories: 310
- Fat: 27g
- Carbohydrates: 7.6g
- Protein: 4.4g
- Dietary Fiber: 1.3g

Lightly Sweet Chocolate Brownie Drops

(Prepping time: 15 mins\ Cooking time: 10 mins |For 12 servings)

Another recipe for the chocolate tooth out there who are looking for a nice and tasty treat filled with the sensuous flavor of chocolate! Batch up these brownie drops which are both healthy and sweet!

Ingredients:

- 1/8 cup of stone ground whole wheat pastry flour
- 2 tablespoon of Whole grain soy flour
- ¼ teaspoon of Baking Powder
- 3 ounce of Unsweetened Baking Chocolate Squares
- 6 tablespoon of Heavy Cream
- 2 tablespoon of Unsalted Butter Stick
- 2 large sized whole egg
- 3/4 cup of sucralose based Sweetener

Preparation:

1) The first step here is to pre-heat your oven to a temperature of 375 degree Fahrenheit while lining up your baking sheet with a fine parchment paper
2) Take a big bowl and whisk in your 2 tablespoon of flour alongside baking powder and soy flour
3) Take an oven proof bowl and put your chocolate and butter and cream on it. Place it in your microwave for about 120 seconds until the chocolate is tender and butter is softened
4) Leave it standing for about 120seconds and stir it until very smooth
5) Using an electric mixer, you are going to want to beat up your sugar substitute and eggs until a nice light & fluffy texture has been achieved. It should not take more than 3 minutes
6) Then finely beat up your warm chocolate mix into that egg mix and blend again for 1 minutes making sure to turn down the mixer speed to low, while mixing the flour as well

7) Take a rounded spoon and keep dropping the batter onto your prepared baking sheet until all mixture is used up
8) Bake for about 5-6 minutes and transfer to the wired rack to nicely cool it up

Nutrition Values

- Calories: 104
- Fat: 9.4g
- Carbohydrates: 3.9g
- Protein: 2.5g
- Dietary Fiber: 3.9g

Unexpectedly Baked Pear Fan

(Prepping time: 10 minutes\ Cooking time: 40 minutes |For 4 servings)

Yet another Pear recipe, but this a bit more unique one. That is why the title has "unexpected" in it. But don't worry though! While this might look weird, you will most definitely love the combination of pear, pepper, ginger and cinnamon going on here!

Ingredients:

- 2 medium sized pears
- 1 tablespoon of Unsalted Butter Stick
- ¼ teaspoon of Black Pepper
- ¼ teaspoon of Ginger
- ¼ teaspoon of Cinnamon
- 1 FL ounce of Tap Water
- ¼ teaspoon of Vanilla Extract

Preparation:

1) The first step here is to pre-heat your oven to a temperature of 375 degree Fahrenheit

2) Next, go ahead and make your pear fans and making ¼ inch slices along the length of your half pear, making sure to start from 1/3 inch from the stem while cutting them all the way down to the bottom

3) Take a baking dish and place your butter to melt it over medium level heat, pour in the lemon juice then alongside ginger, pepper, cinnamon as well as water only to mix it properly

4) After that, take you processed pears and place them on top of your pan

5) Cover it up nicely with aluminum foil and keep baking it until the pears and finely tender, it should take about 40 minutes in total. Make sure to turn the pears over halfway

6) Take a slotted spoon now and transfer the prepared halves and place them on serving plates

7) Gently stir your vanilla into the sauce pan and place it on top of your stove and cook it over medium level heat only to gently reduce the heat after 1 minute

8) Scoop up the sauce all over your pears and serve warmly

Nutrition Values

- Calories: 80
- Fat: 3g
- Carbohydrates: 11.5g
- Protein: 0.4g
- Dietary Fiber: 2.9g

Chocolaty Chocolate Cream Frosty

(Prepping time: 3 minutes\ Cooking time: 0 minutes |For 1 servings)

If you are not in the mood for something heavy, then just freeze up a chilled chocolate frosty to give yourself an ice cream headache while satisfying your flavor palette.

Ingredients:

- ½ cup of tap water
- 2 tablespoon of heavy cream
- 2 tablespoon of sugar free chocolate syrup

Preparation:

1) Here you are going to need to take blender and toss in your cream, syrup, ice cubes and water and blend it until a nice froth appears
2) Sip it up cold

Nutrition Values

- Calories: 119
- Fat: 11.1g
- Carbohydrates: 0.8g
- Protein: 1.6g
- Dietary Fiber: 1g

Melty Ginger Flan

(Prepping time: 180 minutes\ Cooking time: 25 minutes |For 6 servings)

This is more akin to a nice and tasty pudding. But unlike traditional pudding, this won't only give you a sweet taste but also a sensation of spice thanks to the ginger included here! A funky combination to say the least.

Ingredients:

- 3 large side yolks
- 2 large sized whole egg
- 1 and a ½ cups of heavy cream
- 1 cup of tap water
- 8 packets of sucralose based sweetener
- 1 teaspoon of vanilla extract
- 3 teaspoon of ginger

Preparation:

1) The first step here is to pre-heat your oven to a temperature of 350 degree Fahrenheit

2) Gently place a roasting pan on the center shelf of your oven and fill it up about to half with water that is at boiling temperature

3) Take a blender then and toss in the egg, yolk, water, cream, sugar substitute, ginger, vanilla and blend them until smoothened completely

4) Take a sieve and pour the batter through it into a shallow leveled 1 quart baking dish

5) Gently place the dish in a roasting pan in your roasting pan and bake for about 30-35 minutes

6) Then finely transfer it to a cooling rack

7) Once cooled, take a plastic wrap and spray it with cooking spray . then gently place it over the flan and chill in the fridge for 3 hours

8) Once done, remove the plastic wrap and gently bring out the chilled meal from the container by inverting it over a plat and tapping on the back

9) Eat

Nutrition Values

- Calories: 265
- Fat: 26g
- Carbohydrates: 3.9g
- Protein: 4.6g
- Dietary Fiber: 0g

Chapter 7:
Amazing
Dinner

Tender Baked Tamari Lemon Pork Chops

(Prepping time: 15 minutes | Cooking time: 40 minutes | For 4 servings)

Dinner time is a good family time, possibly the last meal of the day. So why not make something which the whole family can enjoy? This Tender Baked Tamari Lemon Pork Chop will not only fill up your Atkins belly, but also the belly of your family members!

Ingredients:

- 8 tablespoon of Tamari Soybean Sauce
- 2 tablespoon of Worcestershire Sauce
- 2 teaspoon of Garlic
- 1 FL ounce of fresh lemon juice
- 1 teaspoon Canola Vegetable Oil
- ½ a teaspoon of Black Pepper
- 1 and a ½ pound of Pork Chop with Center Loin and Bone-In

Preparation:

1) Take a shallow dish and toss in the tamari, minced up garlic, Worcestershire sauce, pepper, lemon juice and the oil only to mix them properly
2) Toss in the pork chops in that mixture then and coat it finely
3) Cover it up and let it freeze in your refrigerator for about 1 hour
4) Pre-heat your oven to a temperature of 375 degree Fahrenheit
5) Once done, remove the chops their marinade and dry them up
6) Place them in your roasting pan and bake for about 35-40 minutes or so
7) Once done, take them out and serve

Nutrition Values

- Calories: 149
- Fat: 8
- Carbohydrates: 4g
- Protein: 15.2g
- Dietary Fiber: 0.1g

Dreamy Cali Mac and Cheese

(Prepping time: 15 minutes\ Cooking time: 20 minutes |For 6 servings)

Perhaps one of the most painful restriction of Atkins is not being able to swallow up Pasta or noodles. This recipe is designed to save you from the horror by giving you something that is equally as tasty as mac and cheese, but perfectly suitable with your Atkins diet.

Ingredients:

- 1 large cauliflower head
- 1 cup of heavy cream
- 2 ounce of cream cheese
- 1 and a ½ teaspoon of Mustard
- 1 and a ½ cup of shredded cheddar cheese
- 1 clove of garlic
- 1 teaspoon of salt
- ¼ teaspoon of white pepper
- ¼ teaspoon of original pepper sauce

Preparation:

1) The first step here is to pre-heat your oven to a temperature of 375 degree Fahrenheit
2) Take a baking dish and prepare it nicely with olive oil spray
3) Take a large pot over your stove and fill it up with water only to bring it to a boil
4) Toss in about ½ a teaspoon of salt
5) Gently remove the stem and leave off your cauliflower head and cut into small sized florets
6) Toss them in the boiling water and cook for about 5 minutes until nicely crisp tender
7) Drain it out and pat them in kitchen towel to dry
8) Take a medium sized sauce pan and pour in your cream, only to bring it to a simmer
9) After which, whisk in the cream cheese alongside powdered mustard sauce until nicely smooth
10)   Toss in the shredded cheddar, ½ a teaspoon of salt, minced up garlic, pepper

sauce, white pepper and keep whisking until the whole cheese has melted
11) Turn the heat off and keep stirring the cauliflower
12)   Once done, pour the mixture into your baking dish and top it up with ½ a cup of cheese and bake for 15 minutes until nicely browned

Nutrition Values

- Calories: 320
- Fat: 27
- Carbohydrates: 5.6g
- Protein: 11.4g
- Dietary Fiber: 3.6g

Tantalizing Cheddar Omelet With Avocado And Salsa

(Prepping time: 15 minutes\ Cooking time: 20 minutes |For 6 servings)

Care to end your day just the way you started your day? This vegetable filled omelet is what you want! Taking care of your Atkins diet in style.

Ingredients:

- 1 teaspoon of Canola Vegetable Oil
- 2 large sized whole egg
- 1 ounce of cheddar cheese
- ½ a fruit of deseeded and skinned California avocado
- 1 ounce of Salsa

Preparation:

1) The first step here is to heat up your skillet over medium heat
2) Toss in your lightly beaten egg and cook for 3 minutes

3) Once done, flip them over and cook the other side for 2 minutes more
4) Toss in your shredded cheddar and avocado alongside half portion of the omelet
5) Fold the omelet
6) Let it cook for another 1 minutes to allow the cheese to melt
7) Top everything up with a good amount of salsa and serve hot

Nutrition Values

- Calories: 419
- Fat: 33.6g
- Carbohydrates: 5.2g
- Protein: 20.8g
- Dietary Fiber: 5g

A Pudding From Yorkshire

(Prepping time: 5 minutes\ Cooking time: 35 minutes |For 9 servings)

Yorkshire puddings are a kind of staple for Englishmen. And if you are one of them or you want to try out how English people end their Atkins day! Try this pudding recipe straight out of Yorkshire.

Ingredients:

- ½ a cup of Whole Grain Soy Flour
- 2 ounce of Vital Wheat Gluten
- 3 large sized whole egg
- 1 cup of whole milk
- 1 teaspoon of Salt
- 1 /3 cup of Canola Vegetable Oil
- 1 teaspoon of Baking Powder

Preparation:

1) The first step here is to pre-heat your oven to a temperature of 450 degree Fahrenheit

2) Take a bowl and whisk up your gluten, soy flour, eggs, salt and milk
3) Take an 8 inch square baking dish and pour some oil in it
4) Gently place the baking dish on the center rack of your oven and wait for about 5 minutes
5) Once the oil is smoking hot, pour in your batter and bake for 15 minutes
6) Lower down your temperature to 350 degree Fahrenheit and bake it for another 15-20 minutes until it is showing a lightly brown texture.
7) Serve hot

Nutrition Values

- Calories: 157
- Fat: 11.8g
- Carbohydrates: 3.8g
- Protein: 9.2g
- Dietary Fiber: 0.5g

Spicy Red Bell Pepper Filled Up With Cherry Tomatoes and Feta

(Prepping time: 10 minutes\ Cooking time: 45 minutes |For 4 servings)

These mini tomatoes are filled up with feta cheese to make these nothing short of miniature pizza bombs!

Ingredients:

- 2 medium sized sweet red pepper
- 2 ounce of feta cheese
- 8 pieces of cherry tomatoes
- ½ a teaspoon of ground thyme
- 2 tablespoon of basil
- 1 tablespoon of Extra Virgin Olive Oil

Preparation:

1) The first step here is to pre-heat you oven to a temperature of 400 degree Fahrenheit
2) Take you pepper and cut them into half int lengthwise direction.

3) Gently remove the stem, seeds and ribs of the pepper
4) Take a bowl and toss in your tomatoes, feta, basil and thyme and mix them finely
5) Fill up your pepper halves with the prepared mixture
6) Take a baking dish and drizzle it all over with oil
7) Cover it with aluminum foil and bake it for about 30 minutes
8) Remove the foil then and bake for another 15 minutes until the tomatoes burst out and the cheese has a golden brown texture.

Nutrition Values

- Calories: 97
- Fat: 6.8g
- Carbohydrates: 4.6g
- Protein: 3.2g
- Dietary Fiber: 1.9g

A Healthy Dose of Braised Leeks and Fennel

(Prepping time: 15 minutes \ Cooking time: 45 minutes |For 8 servings)

Leeks and Fennel on their own might seem ordinary. But braise them up with chicken broth, and will get something entirely different and unique! A healthy dose for your flavor palette indeed.

Ingredients:

- 4 pieces of Leeks
- 1 Fennel bulb
- 1 cup of Chicken Broth
- 1 teaspoon of Salt
- ½ teaspoon of Black Pepper
- 3 tablespoon of Unsalted Butter Stick
- 1 tablespoon of Fresh Lemon Juice
- 1/3 cup of Parsley

Preparation:

1) Start off this recipe by pre-heating your oven to a temperature of 450 degree Fahrenheit
2) Take a 11 inch by 9 inch pan and pour in your broth, leeks, fennel and sprinkle pepper and salt
3) Dot it up with butter and cover up the pan with an aluminum foil
4) Bake it for about 15 minutes
5) Once done, pull off the aluminum foil and stir it lightly until the vegetables are nicely tender
6) Pour in your lemon juice alongside the parsley and serve

Nutrition Values

- Calories: 77
- Fat: 4.6g
- Carbohydrates: 7.1g
- Protein: 1.3g
- Dietary Fiber: 1.8g

Completely Browned Up Pumpkin With Maple And Sage

(Prepping time: 10 minutes\ Cooking time: 15 minutes |For 8 servings)

While there are many people who don't like pumpkin these days, doesn't mean that you should avoid them as well! Pumpkins are naturally pretty good tasting, but once you brown them up with a combination of maple and sage, you will have an irresistible Pumpkin delight.

Ingredients:

- 1 pound of Pumpkin
- ¼ cup of chopped up shallots
- 1 tablespoon of unsalted butter stick
- ¼ cup of bouillon vegetable broth
- 1/1 cup of sugar free syrup
- ¼ teaspoon of ground sage

Preparation:

1) The first step here is to take a medium sized skillet and keep it over medium

high heat. Toss in the butter and let it melt

2) In the mean-time, cube up your pumpkin into ¾ inch chunks

3) Toss in the shallots alongside the pumpkins to the pan and season it with freshly ground pepper and salt

4) Sauté it for about 8-10 minutes until the pumpkin is slightly browned up and the shallots are showing a translucent texture

5) Pour in the maple syrup and toss the sage, making sure to combine them nicely

6) Serve hot

Nutrition Values

- Calories: 26
- Fat: 1.2g
- Carbohydrates: 3.5g
- Protein: 0.6g
- Dietary Fiber: 0.4g

The Hottest Buffalo Hot Wing Cauliflower

(Prepping time: 10 minutes\ Cooking time: 45 minutes |For 4 servings)

This is a very classical way of feeding cauliflower to kids who don't like to eat vegetables. Are you one of them? Well, batch up this recipe and it should make your Atkins recipe just as easier to follow! With just the right amount of spicy tanginess.

Ingredients:

- 1 large head of cauliflower
- 2 tablespoon of light olive oil
- 4 tablespoon of Red Hot Buffalo Wing Sauce
- 3 teaspoon of Sriracha Hot Chili Sauce
- 2 tablespoon of Unsalted Butter Stick
- 1 and a ½ ounce of Blue cheese

Preparation:

1) Start off by pre-heating your oven to a temperature of 375 degree Fahrenheit
2) Take your cauliflower head and cut it up into small sized florets
3) Drizzle them up with about 1 tablespoon of olive oil
4) Take a baking sheet and roast them for 35-40 minutes
5) In the meantime, take a small sized sauce pan and pour in the sriracha and hot wing sauce and heat them for 10 minutes until a boiling point is reached
6) Toss in the butter until and keep stirring it until the butter is fully molten
7) Let it cool until it reaches room temperature
8) Toss in the roasted cauliflower and sauté them for about 1 minute and pour in the hot sauce and keep continuing for another minute.
9) Keep tossing it to make sure that the flowers are fully coated.
10) Serve hot with blue cheese sprinkled up on top of the cauliflowers

Nutrition Values

- Calories: 177
- Fat: 14.9g
- Carbohydrates: 4.1g
- Protein: 5.3g
- Dietary Fiber: 4.2g

Conclusion

Once again, I would like you to thank you for downloading this book and having the patience for going through it.

I do hope that you had just as much fun reading and experimenting the meals as much I enjoyed writing the book.

From now on, all you are going to need to do is properly follow the rules of Atkins and go ahead to experiment with your very own meal plan!

Stay safe, Stay healthy and God Bless!

Made in the USA
Columbia, SC
26 September 2017